5-MINUTE RESTORATIVE YOGA STRETCHES FOR SENIORS OVER 60

Gentle Relaxing Exercises to Target Stress, Anxiety, Insomnia, and Joint Pain

NOKO YOGA

Protopian Press

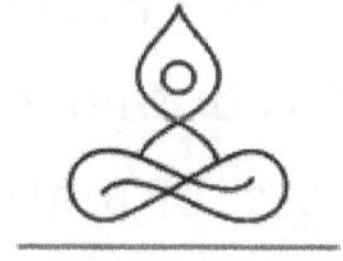

LEGAL NOTICE

DISCLAIMER

The information provided in this book is for educational purposes only. All efforts have been made to present accurate, up-to-date, reliable, and complete information at the time of its publication. However, no warranties of any kind are declared or implied. By purchasing or reading this book, readers acknowledge that the author is not engaged in rendering legal, financial, medical, or professional advice. Please consult a licensed medical professional before attempting any techniques outlined in this book.

By reading this document, the reader agrees that, under no circumstances, is the author responsible for any losses, direct or indirect, that are incurred as a result of the use of the information contained within this document, including, but not limited to, omissions, errors, or inaccuracies. Under no circumstance will any blame or legal responsibility be held against the publisher or author for any damages, repatriation, reparation, or monetary loss due to the information contained within this book, either directly or indirectly. Furthermore, by using this book, you acknowledge that the exercises included in this publication are not without risks of injury or aggravation of preexisting conditions; you agree that you do so at your own risk, assume all risks of injury to yourself, and agree to release and discharge its author, Norkor Omaboe, Daily Cup Of Wellness, from all and any claims or causes of action, known or unknown arising from the author's negligence.

If you begin to experience any physical discomfort at any point, you should stop immediately and consult with a healthcare physician.

LEAVE A REVIEW

If you enjoyed this book, please support me by leaving a review, suggesting it to your friends and family, or offering it as a gift.

To share a review, point your phone's camera at the QR code below and tap the camera on the screen.

OTHER BOOKS BY THE SAME AUTHOR ON AMAZON:

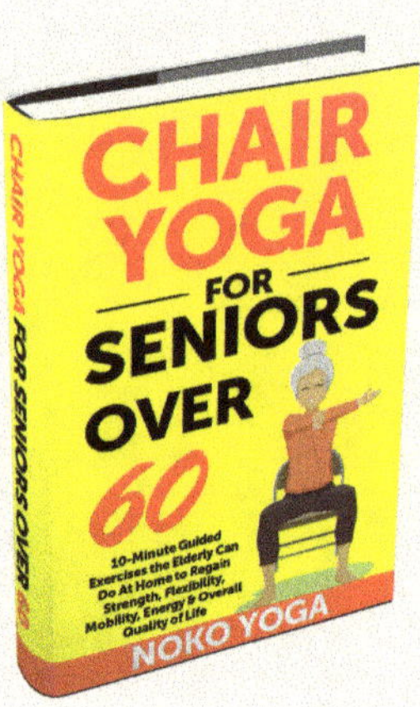

CHAIR YOGA FOR SENIORS OVER 60:

10-Minute Guided Exercises the Elderly Can Do At Home to Regain Strength, Flexibility, Mobility, Energy & Overall Quality of Life

Type the link into your web browser to place your order: https://amzn.to/3MYuoZ9, or point your phone's camera at the QR code below and tap the camera on the screen.

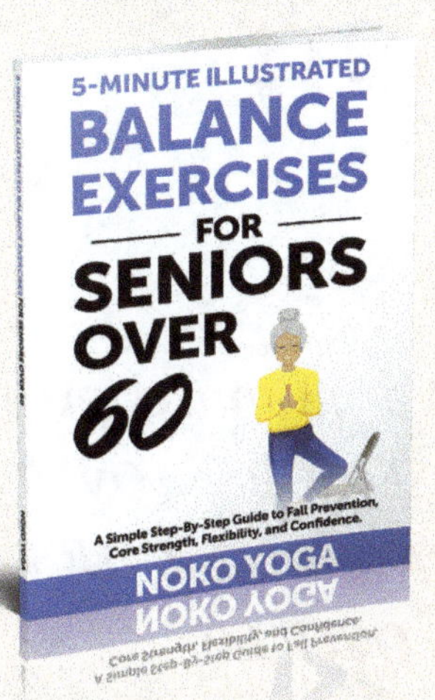

5-MINUTE ILLUSTRATED BALANCE EXERCISES FOR SENIORS OVER 60:

A Simple Step-By-Step Guide to Fall Prevention, Core Strength, Flexibility, and Confidence.

To view the book on Amazon, type the link into your browser, https://amzn.to/3Pd3lvK, or point your phone's camera at the QR code below and tap the camera on the screen.

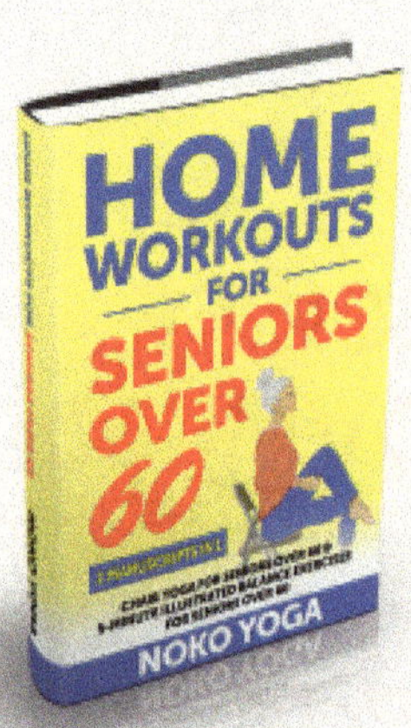

HOME WORKOUTS FOR SENIORS OVER 60:

This book contains two manuscripts, CHAIR YOGA FOR SENIORS OVER 60&5-MINUTE ILLUSTRATED BALANCE EXERCISES FOR SENIORS OVER 60

To view the book on Amazon, type the link into your browser, https://amzn.to/3pmFFea, or point your phone's camera at the QR code below and tap the camera on the screen.

TABLE OF CONTENTS

Unlock the full potential of your wellness journey with personalized training. By seeking individualized guidance, you'll receive a tailored approach and accelerated results. Book a 15-minute FREE Discovery Session with me today by typing the URL in your web browser or by pointing your phone's camera at the QR code and tapping the screen. In this session, we'll go over your struggles, past experiences, goals, and options.

Schedule a FREE session: https://qr1.be/C6CP

Discovery Session QR CODE

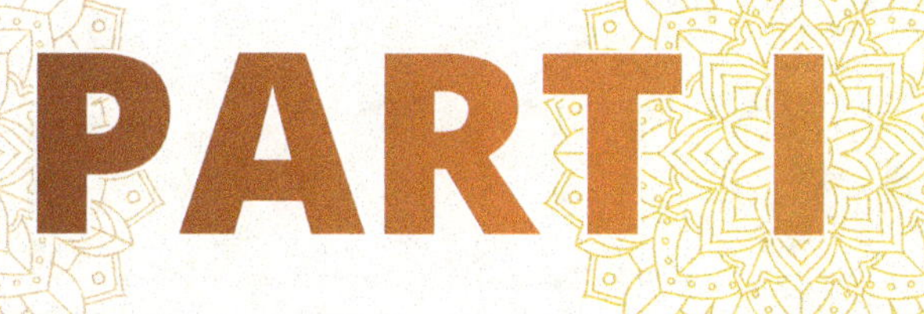

PART I

RESTORATIVE YOGA FUNDAMENTALS

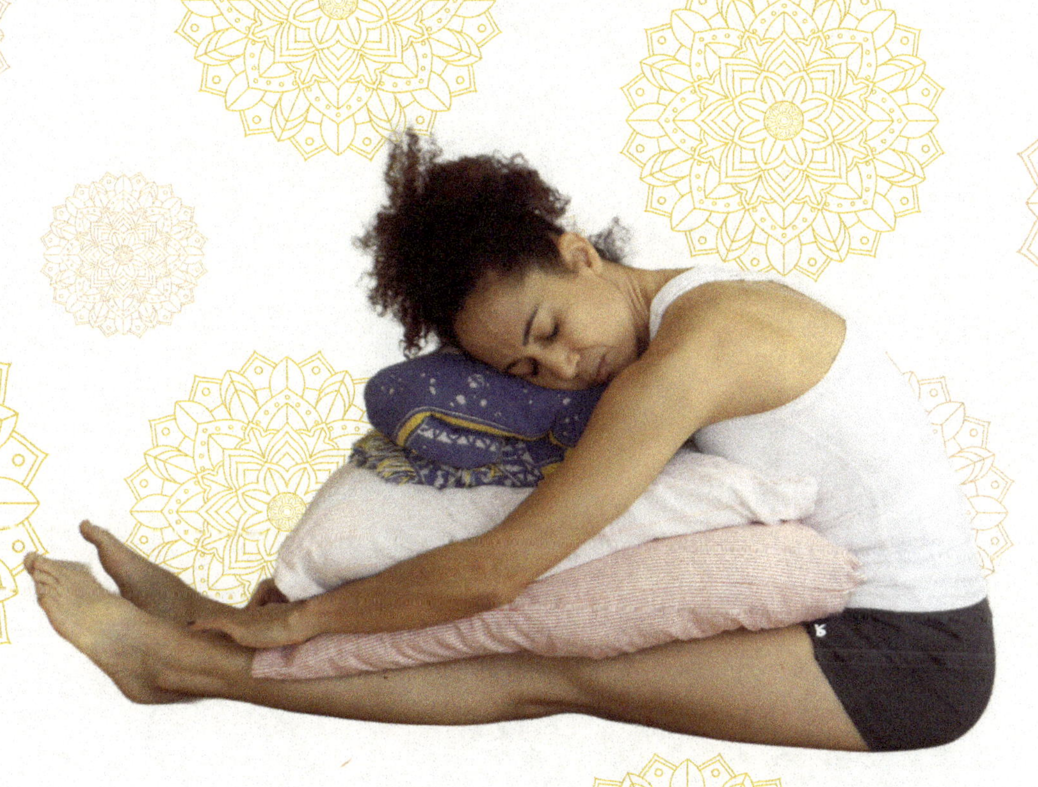

CHAPTER 1

WHAT IS RESTORATIVE YOGA

- Do you ever feel stressed, tense, burnt out, or simply exhausted at the end of a long day?
- Do you need a safe and simple way to unwind and relax from the comfort of your home?
- Does traditional yoga feel out of reach for your painful joints?
- Are you limited by the fear of hurting yourself?

If any of the above questions apply to you, this book can change your life.

Restorative yoga is a gentle form of yoga. Its regenerative aspect allows the body to be supported in all positions, promoting physical and mental relaxation. Research shows that restorative yoga helps reduce symptoms of stress, anxiety, depression, and pain.

Restorative yoga is safe as it can easily be modified to fit your needs and body type. It is about slowing down and letting go. During restorative yoga, your body and mind reset to a meditative state of blissfulness, allowing you to restore and reset your spine and joints and shut off the fight-or-flight responses that cause inflammation and pain.

HOW TO PRACTICE RESTORATIVE YOGA

Your restorative yoga practice can be enhanced by creating a quiet space. Props are an integral part of restorative yoga. Have cushions, bolsters, and blankets available close by. Once in a restorative pose, ensure your neck, lower back, shoulders, and knees are supported. Use your props to cradle your body, inviting relaxation. Start by closing your eyes and connect with your breath. Take deep, slow, conscious breaths, allowing your muscles to release tension. Try to quiet your mind by focusing on your breath and progressively letting your body breathe itself. Enjoy the bliss of each pose for several minutes at first and gradually up to ten minutes. As your muscles relax, adjust the props or modify your posture to feel even more comfortable. Practioners often enhance the experience by dimming the lights, playing soft, soothing music, and diffusing essential oils. Give yourself permission to fully immerse yourself in the moment without expectations. Restorative yoga is a practice that promotes self-care and, when done regularly, produces profound effects on your mind, body, and soul.

HOW TO BREATHE DURING RESTORATIVE YOGA

Conscious breathing is a crucial element of restorative yoga. It keeps your mind in the present moment and deepening the restorative benefits of the practice. As you settle into your position, close your eyes and bring awareness to your breath. Then, take deep, slow inhalations through your nose, allowing your abdomen to rise gently. Notice the cleansing breath fills your lungs. As you exhale, relax even deeper and allow your abdomen to fall naturally. Allow your breath to be effortless and smooth. With each inhalation, invite a sense of relaxation; with each exhalation, let go of thoughts that are not serving you. As you progress through your practice, progressively allow your body to gently breathe itself without trying to control the breath.

CHAPTER 2

BENEFITS OF RESTORATIVE YOGA

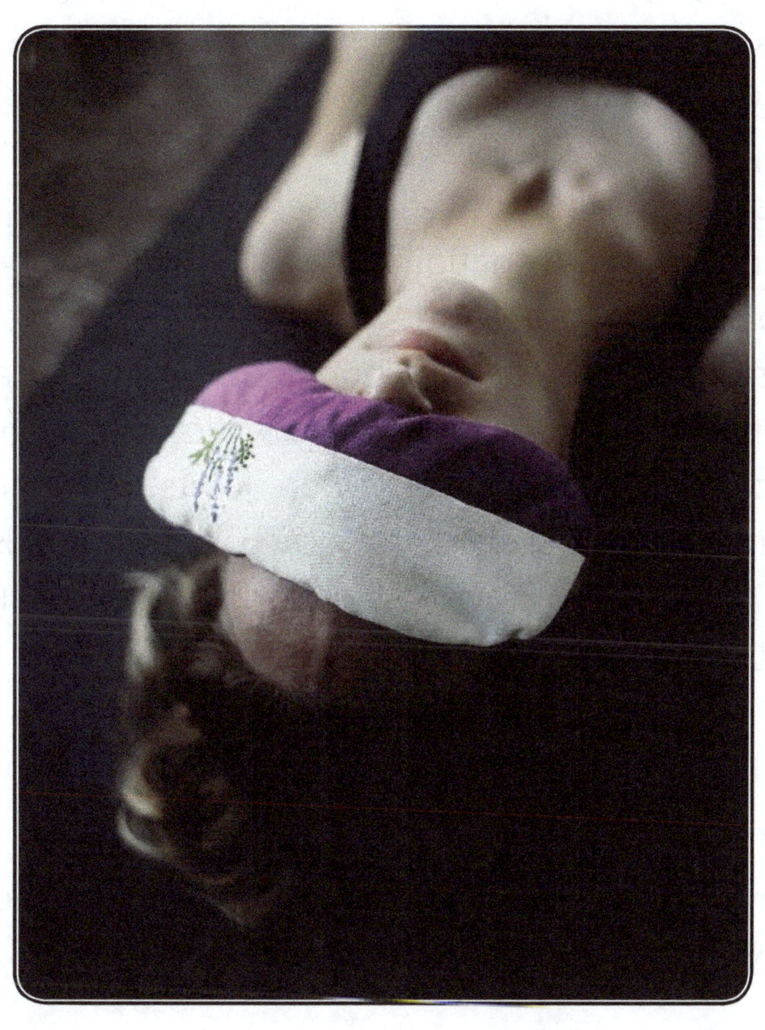

Restorative yoga elicits mental, physical, and spiritual benefits.

RESTORES THE NERVOUS SYSTEM

Restorative yoga elicits a restorative and healing benefit for the nervous system. The stillness of the practice promotes a sense of stillness and calmness; this practice triggers the parasympathetic nervous system. This part of your nervous system is responsible for feeling safe, resulting in profound relaxation and rejuvenation. The slow, conscious breath accompanying each pose shuts off the body's stress responses, known as the fight-or-flight response, and puts your mind and body on pause. You will leave your practice feeling grounded, with a calm energy and renewed joints. This grounding sensation subconsciously signals the brain that it is safe to let go of worries and physical and emotional pain. Practiced regularly, restorative yoga is a vector of healing past traumas.

WEIGHT LOSS

Deep conscious breathing is an integral part of a therapeutic restorative practice. By shutting down the body's fight-or-flight response, restorative yoga helps suppress cortisol. Cortisol is a stress hormone activated during an acute stressor and a protective mechanism. However, because many of us are under chronic stress, excessive stress contributes to fat storage, particularly around the midsection. This type of fat, called visceral fat, does not respond to caloric deficit. Therefore, stress can be the cause of previous weight loss attempts. Incorporating restorative or yin yoga into your daily routine alongside intermittent fasting and regular physical activity will yield much better results. By calming the nervous system, these yoga practices can support your weight loss journey more holistically and comprehensively.

BACK PAIN

Restorative yoga brings transformative relief to those suffering from back and joint pain. Your muscles will lengthen and relax within just a few minutes, offering immediate comfort.

Props, such as folded blankets or bolsters, provide the needed support to the curves of the lower back, neck, and knees. They allow the back muscles to relax and alleviate stiff and tight back muscles fully.

MINDFULNESS

The slow pace of a restorative practice allows you to deepen the experience of each pose, become aware of your sensations, where you might be holding tension, and how your body reacts to each asana (position) without trying to attain a specific goal. This is the perfect opportunity to be in the present, taking pleasure in what is happening moment by moment.

PHYSICAL AND EMOTIONAL TENSION

The supported aspect of restorative yoga allows your joints and muscles to be supported entirely without using any muscular tension. Due to its non-goal-driven aspect, restorative yoga can be practiced without expectations beyond feeling great.

FLEXIBILITY

In restorative yoga, your body is in a gentle, relaxing position for long periods. Props are used to support the poses, making them more comfortable. As the muscle relax into the poses, you can adjust the props and go deeper if you wish. This will have a beneficial effect on flexibility due to the length of time you hold each pose.

MENTAL HEALTH

Restorative yoga quiets the chatter of the mind and offers a moment of stillness in your day. It allows you to disconnect and distance yourself from your busy life. As a result, it reduces stress and anxiety and is a great tool to prepare for sleep.

WHAT YOU CAN EXPECT

As you settle into your positions, it is not uncommon to feel the need to adjust either the position or the props as your muscle relax. Adjusting the props or the position is part of the practice, especially if you are new to restorative yoga.

Note that not all positions work for everybody. Some positions require some level of flexibility. If you find yourself straining or uncomfortable, ease out of the position and select another one for now. Be patient with yourself and understand that it may take time before a particular position feels comfortable.

CHAPTER 3

INTEGRATING RESTORATIVE YOGA INTO YOUR DAILY LIFE

A regular restorative yoga practice provides a physical and emotional escape from the stress of a busy week. This transformative lifestyle provides moments of self-care and promotes physical and mental relief. Start by blocking off a dedicated time in your schedule. Start with a realistic schedule that can be just five minutes of daily practice. The duration and time of your practice can vary from day to day. Some days, your restorative practice can be a brief early morning session to set the tone for the day. On other days, you can have more extended sessions to unwind at the end of a stressful week.

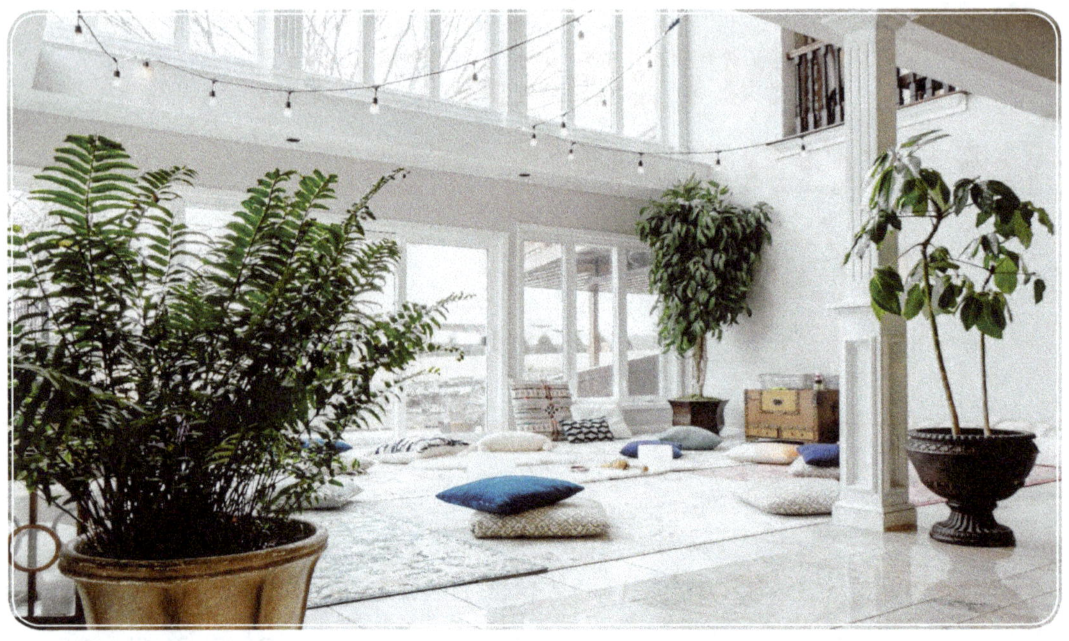

Next, designate a space that promotes tranquility. It can be a peaceful outdoor spot or a corner of your home. Gather all your props, such as blankets, bolsters, and blocks. I like to use a basket that I leave next to my mat.

Take the time to explore poses and variations that suit your body and needs. Aim for at least three to five minutes, and whenever possible, extend the duration to ten to fifteen minutes per pose. As you settle into a pose, you may have to adjust the props to feel supported at all times. If you notice you are straining your muscles, modify the pose or try another. The goal is to feel utterly relaxed and supported. How you move out of the pose is as important as the pose itself. You do not want to undo the benefits of the practice. Take the time to slowly ease out of the position. Slowly ease out of the pose; not all poses are for everybody, and you will find that some require more flexibility. Restorative yoga is not about forcing your body into unrealistic and uncomfortable poses. If you find that you are resisting a pose, simply adjust the position or ease out of the pose.

As you step into this journey, self-love and self-compassion should be your guides. Respect and honor your body's needs, modifying poses as needed. Allow your body to fully surrender to the pose with compassion.

Soon, you will begin to witness a profound transformation from inside out, rippling through the different areas of your life. You will start to let go of thoughts that no longer serve you, become more resilient and focused, and experience reduced joint pain or muscle stiffness.

⚠ WARNING

If you are pregnant or have any medical condition, consult your medical doctor before using this book.

CHAPTER 4

RESTORATIVE YOGA PROPS YOU'LL NEED

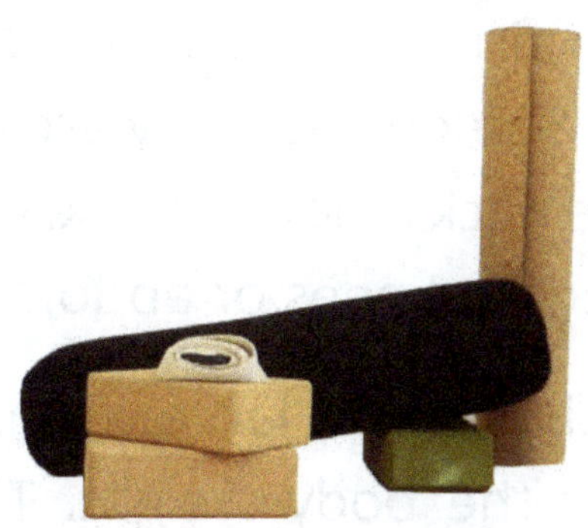

The use of props enhances a traditional restorative yoga practice. However, don't let the lack of props keep you from starting restorative yoga. Yoga props refer to equipment used to support your joints, make the poses more comfortable, and allow your body to remain in the same poses longer.

To learn how to set up your props correctly, request my free video tutorial: **"Restorative Yoga Basic Props Setup."** Copy and paste the link below into your web browser. You will then be redirected to the order form.

Free Video Tutorial: https://bit.ly/46ieX6m

The most common props include:

- Folded blankets of different sizes: I recommend thick cotton blankets over wool blankets because they retain their shape better, providing better support. They provide additional padding between your body and the floor and a cozy feel.
- Pillows and firm cushions of different sizes and thicknesses. Sometimes, they are used to support the arches of the neck or lower back; other times, they are placed under the knees or abdomen.
- Bolsters: Bolsters are large, firm, but soft cushions that support the body weight. They encourage the spine to lengthen, the chest and shoulders to open, and the lower back to relax.

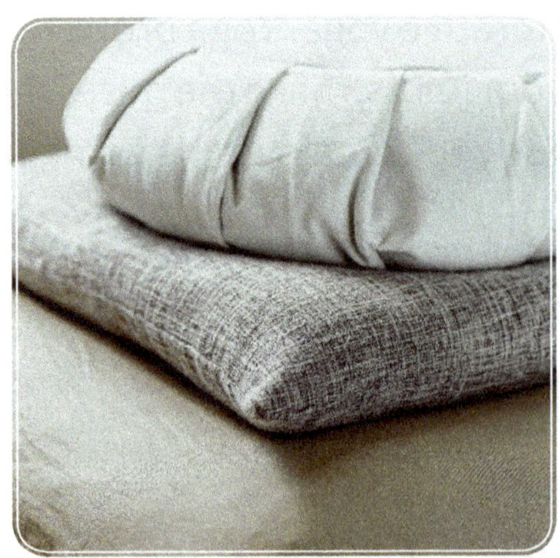

- Blocks: They help modify the position and relieve unnecessary muscle tension and joint strain.

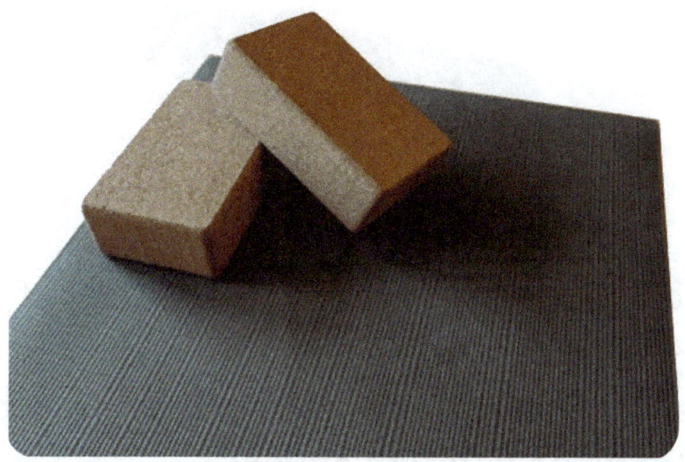

- Yoga straps, belts, or rolled towels
- Eye pillows significantly enhance relaxation by reducing eye and facial strain while blocking light. An alternative is a heating cloth or washcloth. Eye pillows can be used in all supine positions.
- Access to a wall
- A yoga mat or padded surface to lie upon.

BASIC YOGA PROPS SETTINGS

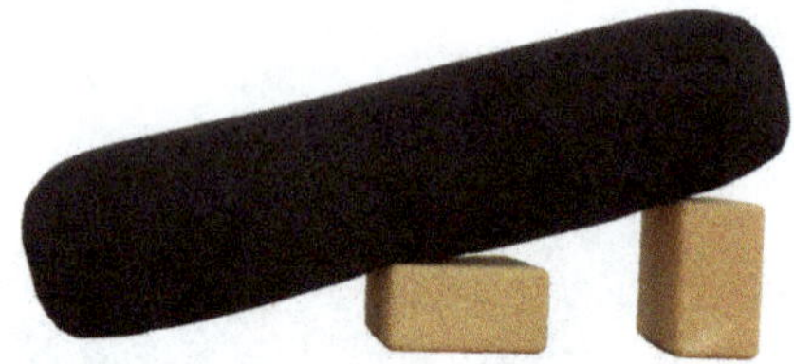

Bolster and blocks: You can shift the side of the blocks depending on the desired incline of your bolster. The incline affects the intensity and/or comfort of the pose, so it's important to try the different options.

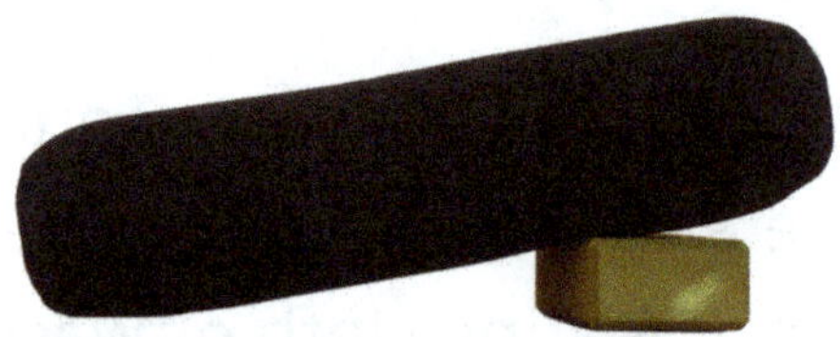

Modify the incline by adding or removing blocks. Books or rolled towels can be used to replace blocks.

CHAPTER 5

TIPS

- Create a restorative yoga practice by setting daily or weekly goals. For example, you can set a reminder on your phone or on a sticky note to remind you to practice just before bedtime. Initially, set your practice with just one exercise for three minutes. Progressively increase the frequency first, then the duration of each pose to meet your needs,
- Set enough time to prep your props and for the full resting time,
- Find a quiet place
- Wear comfortable clothes
- Make sure the room temperature allows you to relax fully. Have an extra blanket to cover yourself if necessary,
- Ease out of the position immediately if you feel any discomfort,

- If you notice you are straining, either modify the position or find a more suitable option,
- Closing your eyes or using an eye pillow will help connect inwards and relax the facial muscles, including the eye muscles,
- Start by practicing deep, slow breathing while resting in your position. Eventually, your body will breathe itself as you fall into deep relaxation,

PART II

RESTORATIVE YOGA POSES

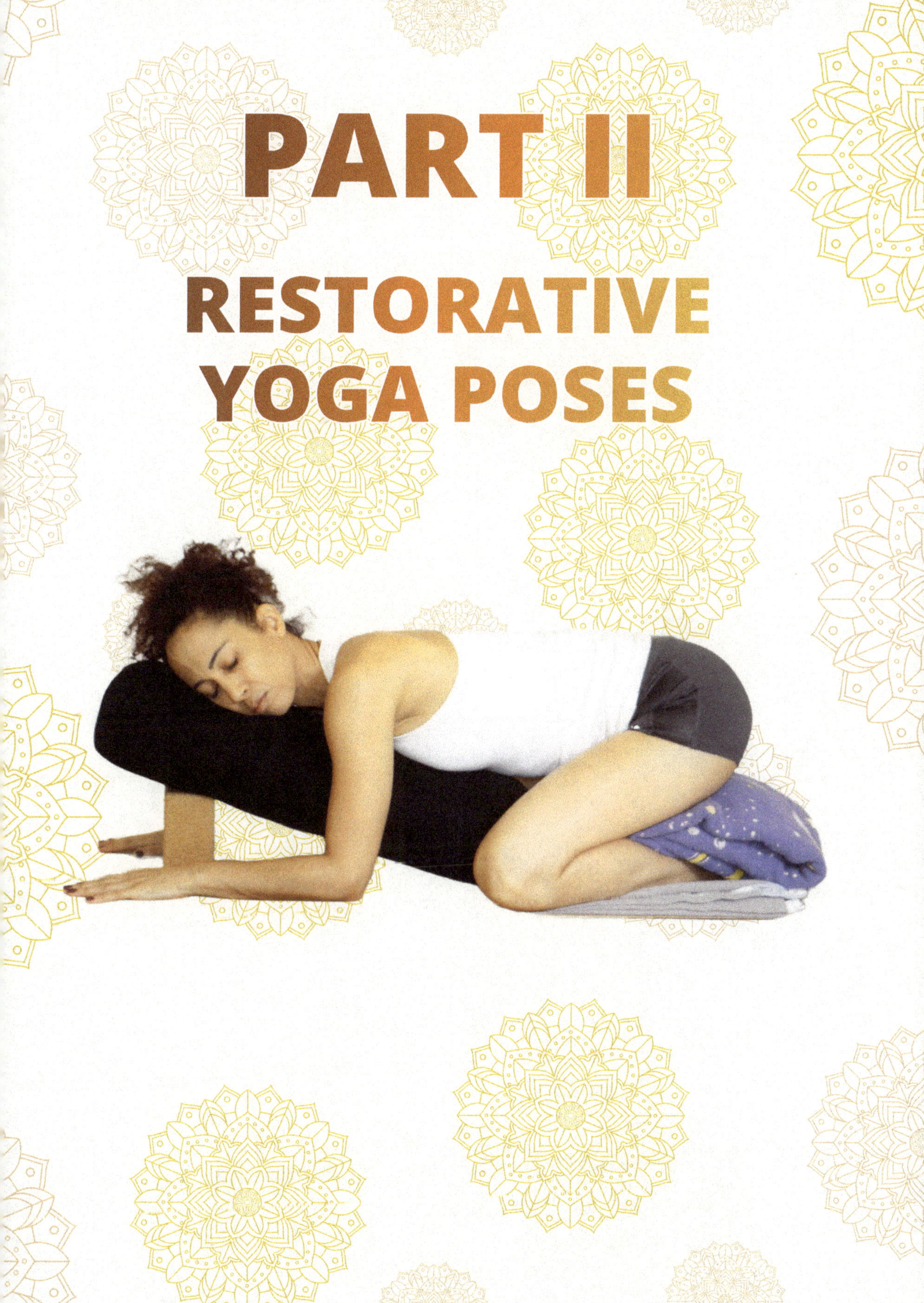

CHAPTER 6

LOWER BACK RELIEF

SUPINE INCLINE POSES

Supine incline poses are a good choice for meditation and breathing exercises.

INCLINED SAVASANA

Variation A: Basic Set Up

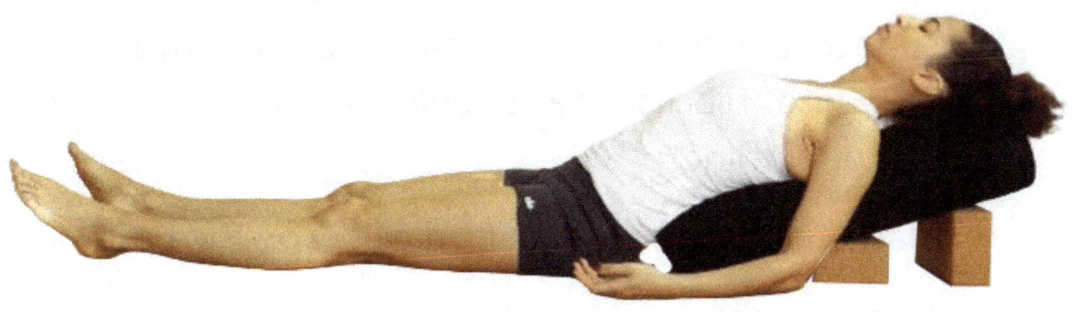

BENEFITS

Savasana is a traditional yoga pose often practiced at the end of a yoga class. It calms the nervous system and reduces stress and muscular tension. Savasana pose helps improve the quality of sleep, reduce stress, and manage blood pressure. Inclined Savasana or Corpse Pose helps relieve tired, achy back, lower back, and neck tension and opens up the chest and shoulders. This variation is particularly beneficial if you experience lower back pressure when lying on your back.

SET UP

- Use two blocks to create the base of the incline
- The block closer to the hips should be laid on its larger surface
- The block further out should be placed on its small surface. Books, pillows, or folded towels may be used instead of blocks. They should be set up to create a smooth incline
- Place a bolster or a large firm pillow on the base
- Close your eyes
- Rest for 5 minutes or longer.

INCLINED SAVASANA

Variation B: supported neck and knees

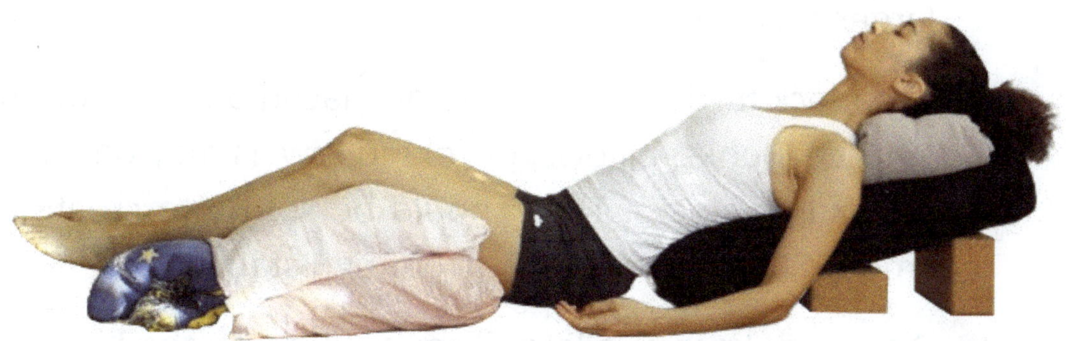

BENEFITS

Savasana calms the nervous system and reduces stress and muscular tension. This restorative pose improves the quality of your sleep and manages blood pressure. Inclined Savasana or Corpse Pose helps relieve tired, achy back, lower back, and neck tension and opens up the chest and shoulders. The rolled towel underneath the neck provides additional support and neck release. The pillows under the knees provide additional benefits to the lower back.

SET UP

- Use two blocks to create the base of the incline
- The block closer to the hips should be placed on its larger surface
- The block further out should be placed on its medium surface. Books, pillows, or folded towels may be used instead of blocks. They should be set up to create a smooth incline and provide enough stability
- Place a bolster or a large firm cushion on the base of the blocks
- Sit up close so that your tailbone is close to the edge of the bolster. The edge of the bolster should provide support for the curve of your lower back
- Fold a small blanket underneath the curve of your neck
- Place a couple of pillows under your knees. This will provide extra relief to your lower back
- Roll a small towel under your ankles so they do not hang off the pillows.
- Close your eyes
- Rest for 5 minutes or longer.

SUPINE HORIZONTAL POSES

SAVASANA WITH SUPPORTED NECK AND KNEES

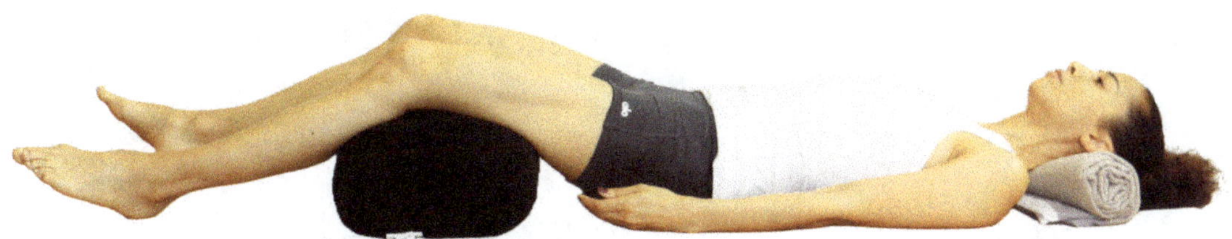

ALTERNATIVE SETTINGS

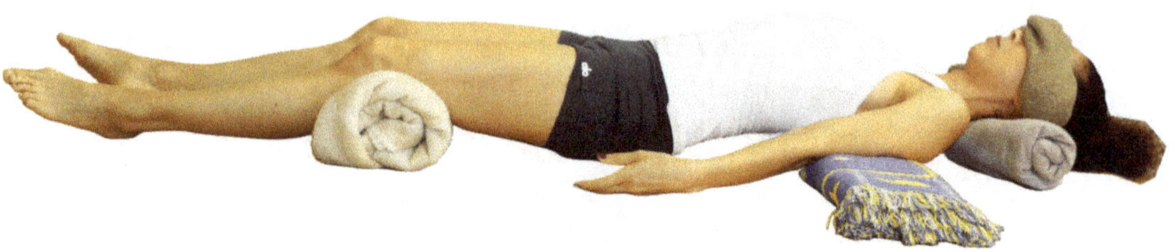

A blanket can be used instead of the bolster underneath the knees. The blanket under the shoulder blades helps open the chest and reduce upper back tightness.

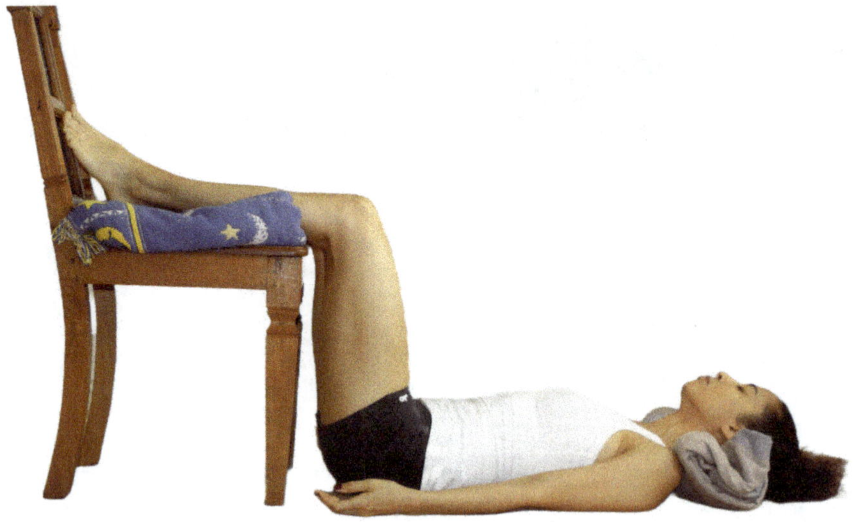

The elevated legs provide additional lower back relief and improve circulation.

BENEFITS

Savasana calms the nervous system and reduces stress and muscular tension. This resting pose helps improve sleep and manage blood pressure. Bending the knees when laying in Savasana takes the pressure off the lower back and allows the thigh muscles to relax fully. The rolled towel under the neck allows the body to feel fully supported and releases muscle tension.

SET UP

- Lay on your back with a rolled towel or bolster underneath your knees. Alternatively, you can rest your legs on a chair.
- Place a rolled towel underneath your neck
- Optional: use an eye pillow to cover your eyes, allowing your body to fall deeper into a restorative state
- Rest for 5 minutes or longer.

SUPPORTED BUTTERFLY

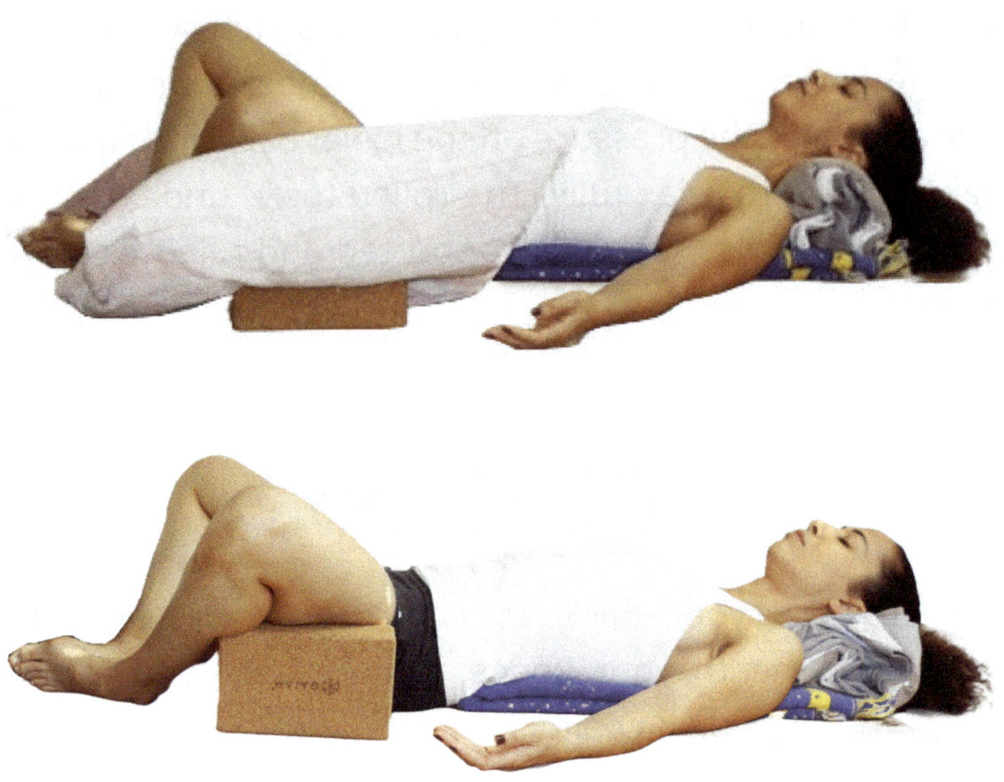

BENEFITS

This pose relaxes the entire body and releases stress, fatigue, anxiety, and muscle tension. It quiets the mind, supports the lower back, and helps reduce lower back tension. Additionally, the butterfly pose opens up the hips.

SET UP

- Fold a blanket lengthwise to provide a soft surface for your spice. Your shoulders should be able to "fall off" the blanket.
- Roll a blanket to fit the curve of your neck. When you lay on your back, your face should face the ceiling.
- Lay on your back with the soles of your feet facing one another, allowing your knees to open.
- Place blocks and pillows underneath your thighs to support your legs. You should be able to relax without inner thigh tension or hip discomfort fully.
- Close your eyes
- Rest for five minutes or longer.

TIPS

The more support underneath your knees, the easier the pose is. If you are holding tension in your inner thighs, add additional pillows under your knees.

SUPINE DECLINE POSES

⚠ WARNING

All decline poses should be avoided during pregnancy, glaucoma, retinal condition, vertigo, high blood pressure, and possibly other chronic conditions. Consult your medical practitioner before attempting any of these poses.

BRIDGE POSE VARIATIONS

Bridge Variation A: Low Supported Bridge Pose

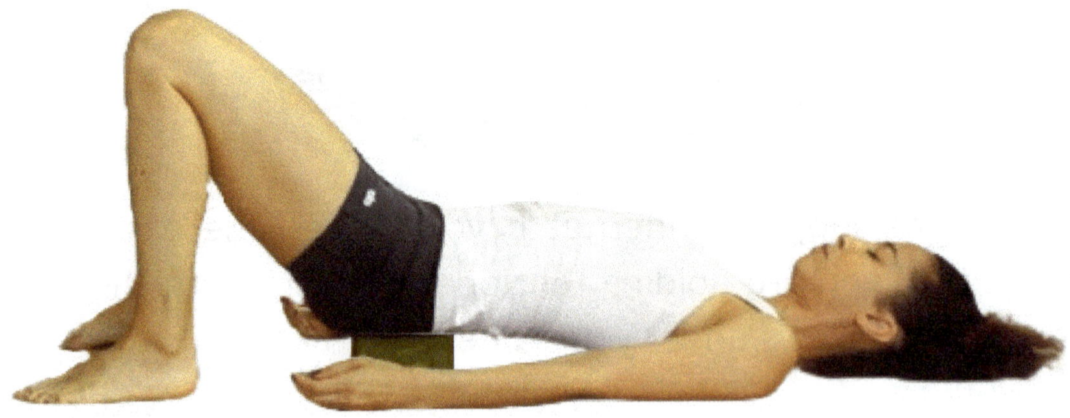

BENEFITS

Restorative Bridge Pose calms the nervous system and restores the lower back posture and alignment from sitting for long hours. This pose helps relieve lower back pain. Bridge Pose also promotes digestion, restores the nervous system, relaxes the tired lower back and legs, helps blood pool into the legs to move back to the heart, and improves oxygen to the brain.

INSTRUCTIONS

- Lay on your back
- Bend your knees
- Lift your hips and place a block on its larger surface underneath your lower back. Keep your tailbone off the block.
- Keep your feet and knees hip-width apart.
- Close your eyes
- Rest for 3-5 minutes.

Bridge Variation B: High Supported Bridge Pose with Eye Pillow

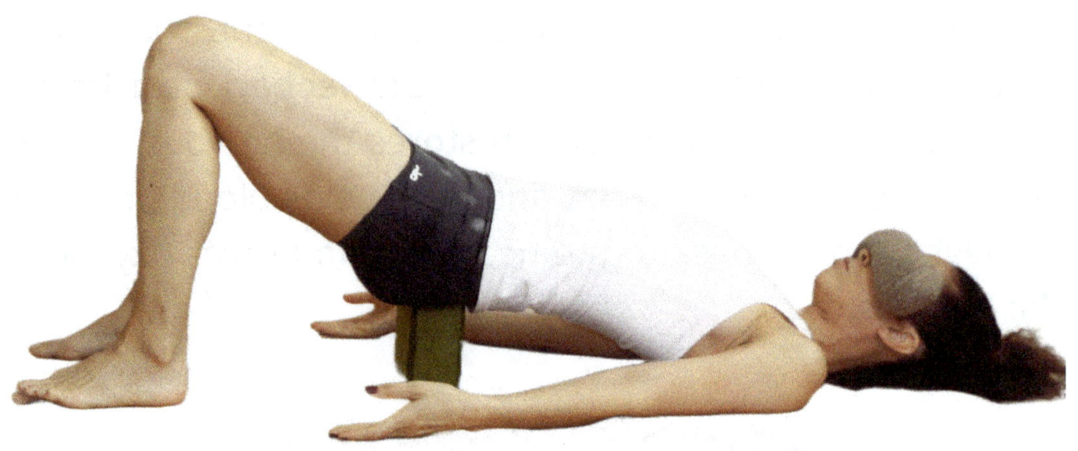

BENEFITS

Restorative Bridge Pose calms the nervous system and improves poor lower back posture and alignment from sitting for long hours. This pose helps relieve lower back pain. This variation is more intense than the Low Supported Bridge Pose.

INSTRUCTIONS

- Lay on your back
- Bend your knees
- Lift your hips and place a block on its small surface underneath your lower back. Keep your tailbone off the block.
- Keep your feet and knees hip-width apart.
- Close your eyes
- Cover your eyes with an eye pillow or wash cloth for additional therapeutic benefits.
- Rest for 3-5 minutes.

CORPS POSES (SAVASANA) WITH LEGS UP

Variation A: Corpse Pose with Legs Up

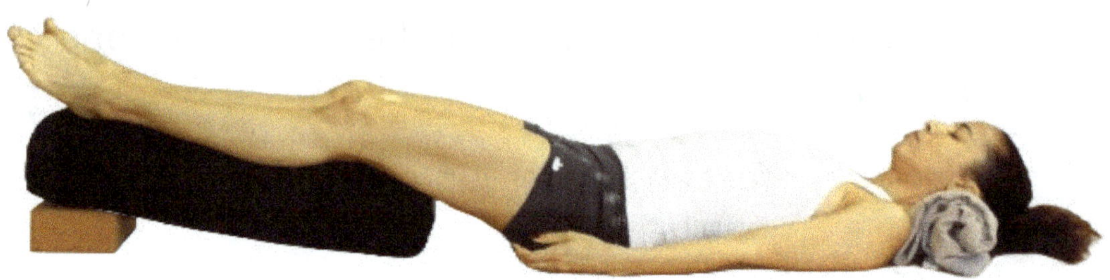

BENEFITS

Corpse Pose, also known as Savasana, helps restore the nervous system, promotes digestion, and improves sleep quality. Savasana with Legs Up relaxes tired legs, helps blood pool into the legs to move back to the heart, and improves oxygen to the brain.

SET UP

- Rest your legs on a bolster or firm pillow. If you do not have a bolster, you may fold layers of blankets and towels to form a decline leg rest.
- Place a block, a book, or a pillow under one end of your bolster.
- Close your eyes
- Relax for five minutes or longer.

TIP

For additional neck relief, roll a towel or small blanket to fill the arch of your neck.

Variation B: Corpse Pose with Supported Legs Up

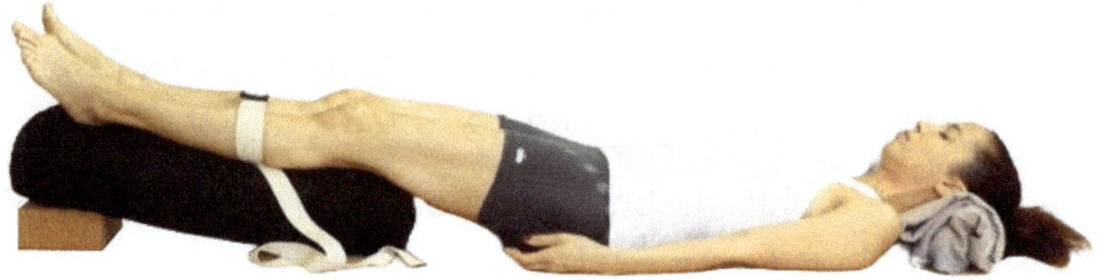

BENEFITS

Corpse Pose, also known as Savasana, helps restore the nervous system, promotes digestion, and improves sleep quality. Savasana with Legs Up relaxes tired legs, helps blood pool into the legs to move back to the heart, and improves oxygen to the brain.

SET UP

- Use a bolster or firm pillow to rest your legs. If you do not have a bolster, you may fold layers of blankets to form a decline leg rest by placing three blankets toward your feet and one folded towel or blanket toward your hips.

- Loosely wrap your legs with a soft strap. This will keep your legs from sliding and falling off the bolster sideways when your muscles surrender to the pose. Next, tie your legs together so there is a small gap between your calves.
- Place a block, book, or pillow under the far end of your bolster.

TIP

For additional neck relief, roll a towel or small blanket to fill the arch of your neck.

LEGS UP AGAINST THE WALL POSES

LEGS UP AGAINST THE WALL WITH KNEES BENT

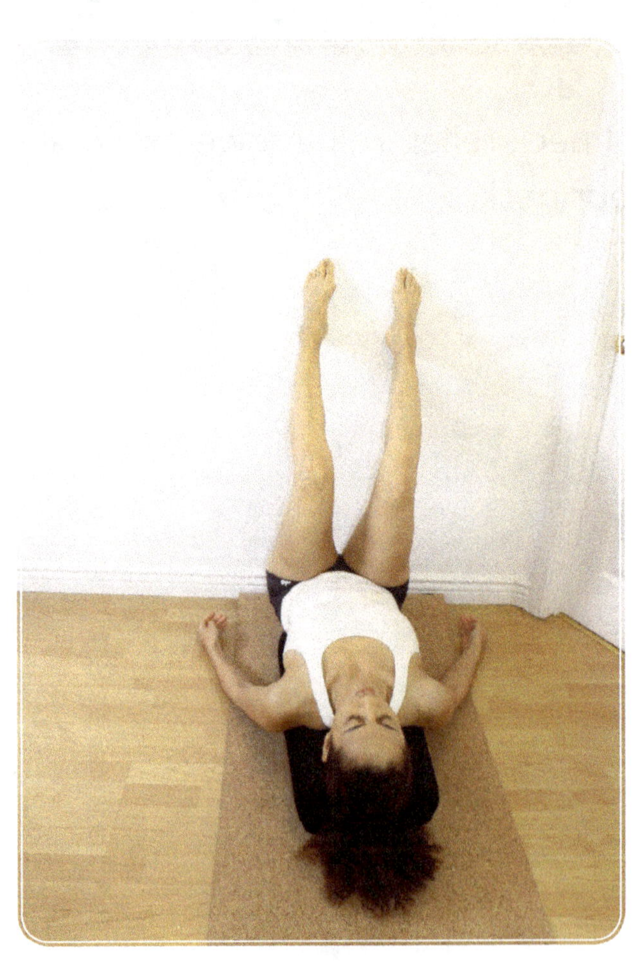

BENEFITS

Leg up-against-the-wall poses reduce lower back strain and muscle tension while reducing blood from pooling into the legs. This pose promotes relaxation and helps reduce the feeling of heavy legs.

SET UP

- Set your bolster about a foot away from a wall
- Lay on your bolster so that the edge of the prop supports your lower back and hips. Keep your tailbone off the bolster. Feel free to adjust the position to make it as comfortable as possible.
- Lift your legs against the wall
- Keep your legs hip-width apart and your knees bent
- Close your eyes
- Relax for 5 minutes or longer.

TIP

Alternatively, you can replace the bolster with a folded towel.

LEG UP AGAINST THE WALL WITH LEG SUPPORT

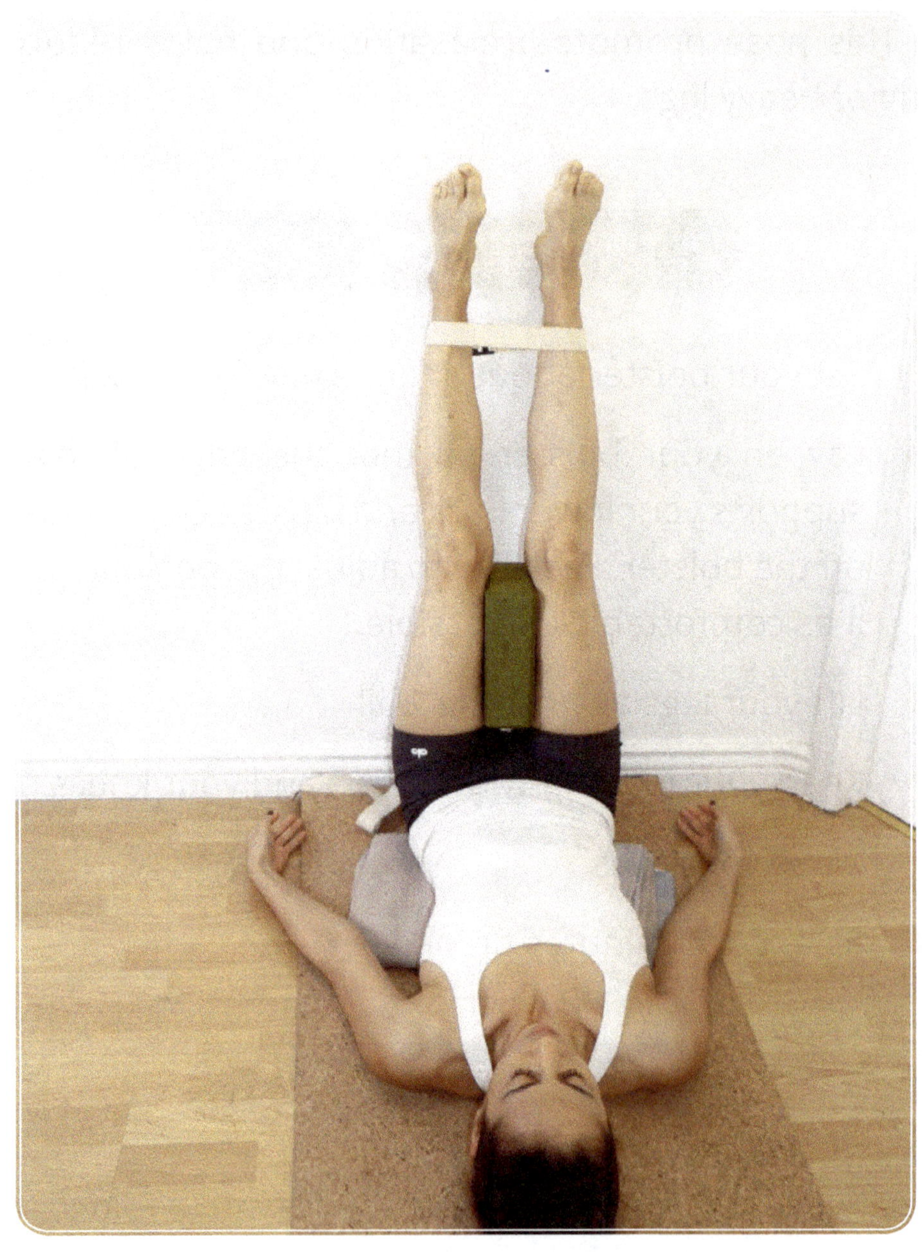

BENEFITS

Legs up against the wall reduce lower back strain and muscle tension and reduce blood from pooling into the legs. It promotes relaxation and helps reduce the feeling of heavy legs. The added props offer more muscle support, allowing the legs to surrender to the pose.

SET UP

- Place a folder blanket about a foot away from a wall
- Sit in front of your folded blanket with your tailbone close to your bolster
- Loosely tie your ankles so that they can rest hip-width apart
- Place a block or pillow between your inner thighs
- Lay on your blanket so that its edge supports your lower back. Feel free to adjust the position of your blanket to make it as comfortable as possible.
- Lift your legs up against the wall
- Close your eyes
- Relax for 5 minutes or longer.

LEGS UP AGAINST THE WALL WITH ARMS AND KNEES EXTENDED

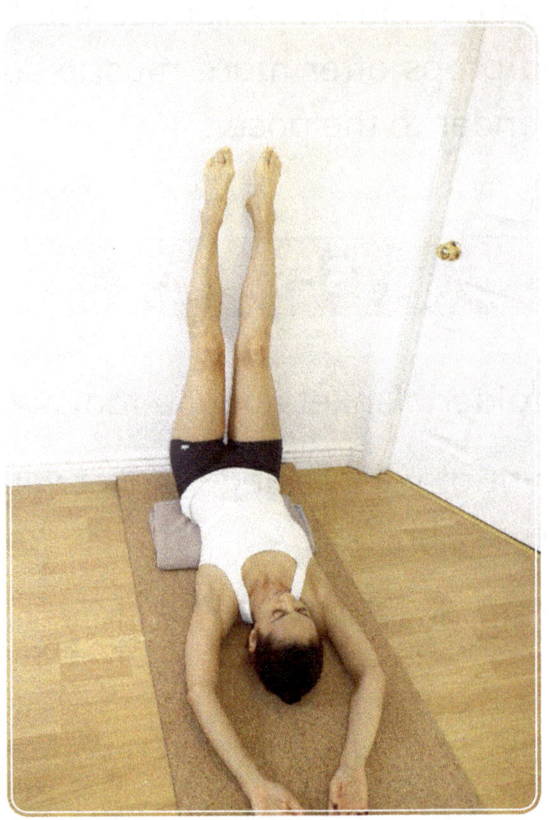

BENEFITS

This variation is best suited for more advanced individuals. The arms above the head help open the chest, upper back, and shoulder stretch. Legs up against the wall reduce lower back strain and muscle tension and prevent blood from pooling into the legs. It promotes relaxation and helps reduce the feeling of heavy legs.

SET UP

- Fold a small blanket on the floor.
- Lay on the blanket so that your tailbone is off the blanket. Adjust the position until you find yourself in a comfortable position. The blanket provides additional support for your lower back, reducing lower back pressure.
- Keep your hips close to the wall
- Extend your legs up against the wall as you lie on your mat
- Extend your arms up for additional upper back and shoulder relief. If this is uncomfortable, open your arms wider and bend your elbows.
- Close your eyes
- Relax for 5 minutes or longer.

BUTTERFLY AGAINST THE WALL

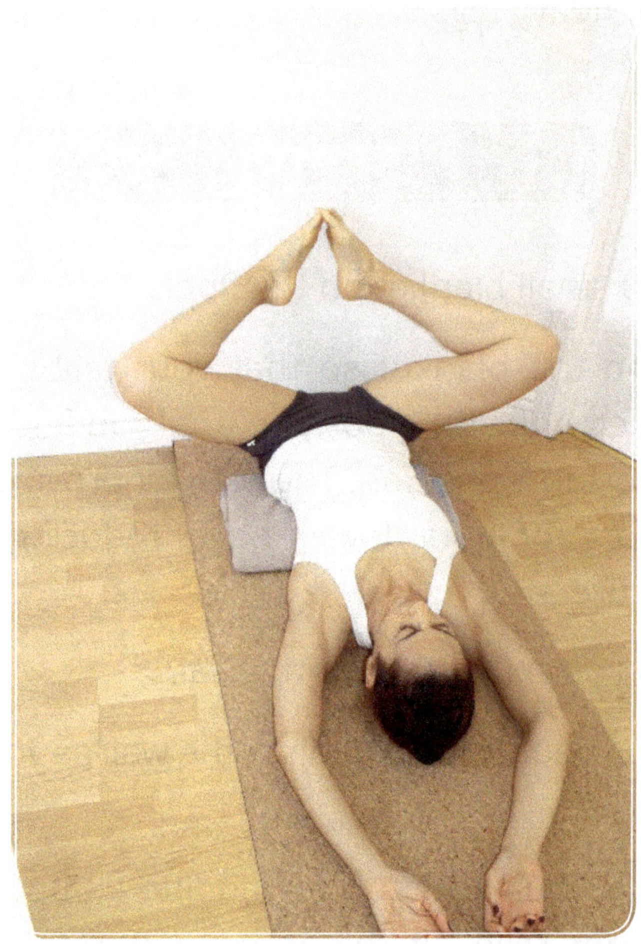

BENEFITS

This position requires some hip flexibility and may not be suitable for a novice practitioner. If you find this pose challenging, scoop your hips away from the wall. Butterfly

Pose against the wall reduces lower back strain and muscle tension and promotes relaxation. This pose opens the hips and stretches the inner thigh muscles. In addition, the arms above the head help open the chest, upper back, and shoulder stretch.

SET UP

- Fold a small blanket on the floor.
- Lay on the blanket so that your tailbone is off the blanket.
- Adjust the position until you find yourself in a comfortable position. The blanket provides additional support for your lower back.
- Lay on your back
- Keep your hips close to the wall as you place your feet against the wall with the sole of your feet against one another.
- Open your knees
- Close your eyes
- Rest for five minutes or longer.

CHAPTER 7

CHILD POSE VARIATIONS

CHILD POSE

INCLINED CHILD POSE

This option is for individuals with limited spine, hips, and knee mobility. Start with this option if you are new to the child pose, as it is less demanding on the joints and muscles. This option provides the most support for your knees, hips, and spine.

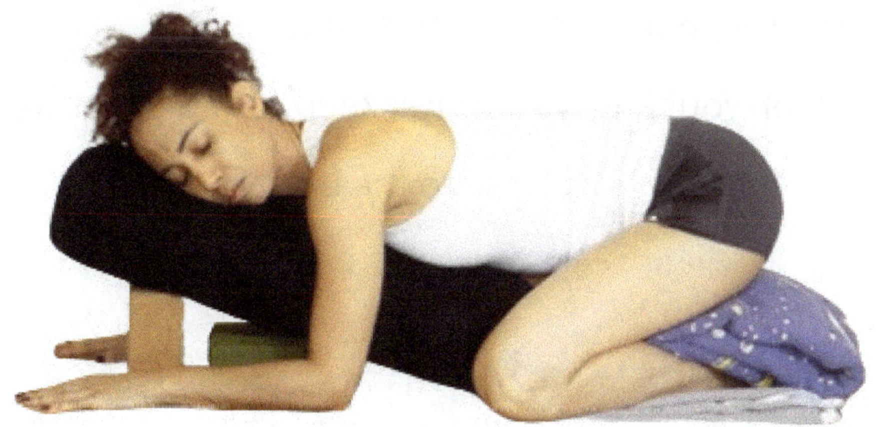

BENEFITS

The child's pose variations calm the mind, relieve stress, open up the hips, stretch the inner thighs, lengthen the lower back muscles and ankles.

SET UP

- Start by setting up your blocks. First, place the block further away on one of its small surfaces to create the incline. Then, place the other block on its large surface.
- Place your bolster over the blocks.
- Fold a blanket to provide padding under your knees.
- Get on all fours with your lower legs on the blanket
- Fold or roll another blanket or large cushion and place it behind your knees. This relieves the knees if you lack the range of motion at this joint.
- Open your knees wide, but keep your big toes together
- Scoop your hips close to the bolster

- Straddle the bolster and lower your hips toward your ankles
- Lay on the bolster and relax for five minutes or longer.

TIP

Add a large pillow at the base of the bolster for extra support. This can be useful if your hips are tight.

Keep your toes tucked under if necessary.

SUPPORTED CHILD POSES

Child Pose with Bolster

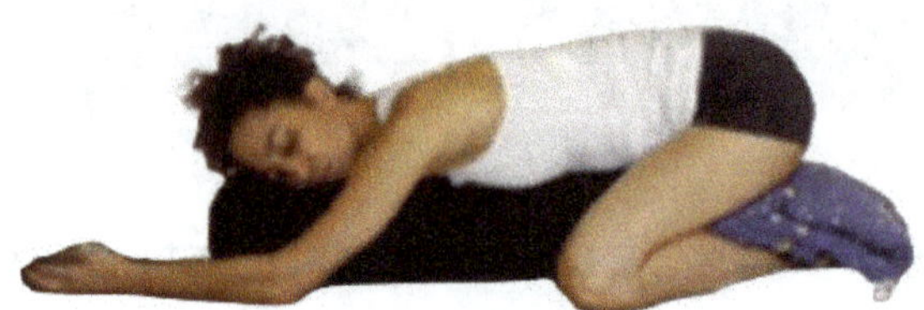

Arms extend forward.

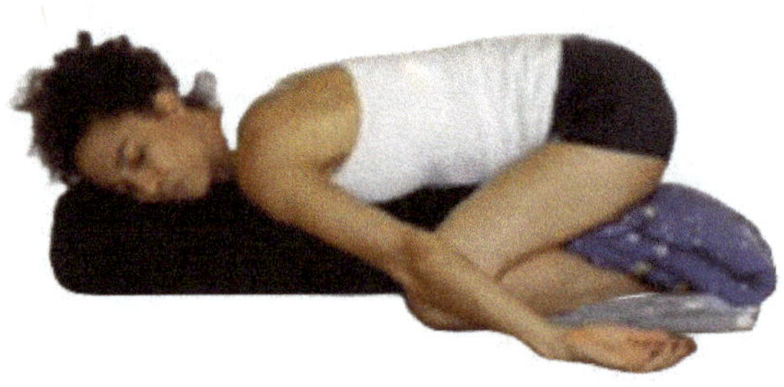

Arms extended toward the feel.

BENEFITS

The child's pose variations calm the mind, relieve stress, open up the hips, stretch the inner thighs, lengthen the lower back muscles, and stretch the ankles. The bolster provides comfort and makes the pose less intense on the hips and lower back.

SET UP

- Place a bolster on your mat
- Get on all fours
- Fold a blanket under your knees for optional padding
- Fold or roll another blanket or pillow and place it behind your knees. If you lack range of motion at this joint, this will relieve the pain.
- Open your knees wide, but keep your big toes together
- Scoop your hips close to the bolster
- Lower your hips toward your heels
- Lay on the bolster or pillows
- Explore extending your arms forward or toward your feet.
- Relax for five minutes or longer.

CHILD POSE WITH BLOCKS

⚠ WARNING

All decline poses should be avoided during pregnancy, glaucoma, retinal condition, vertigo, high blood pressure, and possibly other chronic conditions. Consult your medical practitioner before attempting any of these poses.

These variations are for individuals with limited spine mobility but require moderate hip flexibility. The block slightly elevates the hips to free some range of motion in the knees. The blankets provide support to the knees and elevate the hips.

Experiment with the different head and arms options to determine the most comfortable option.

Variation A: Extended Child Pose with Block

This variation opens and stretches the shoulders. If this is uncomfortable or you have tight shoulders, try variation B.

Variation A: Extended Child's Pose with Block Face Down

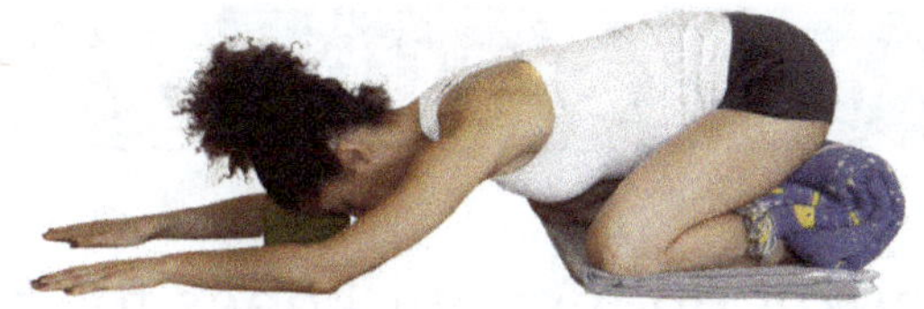

Variation B: Child Pose with Block, head facing sideways

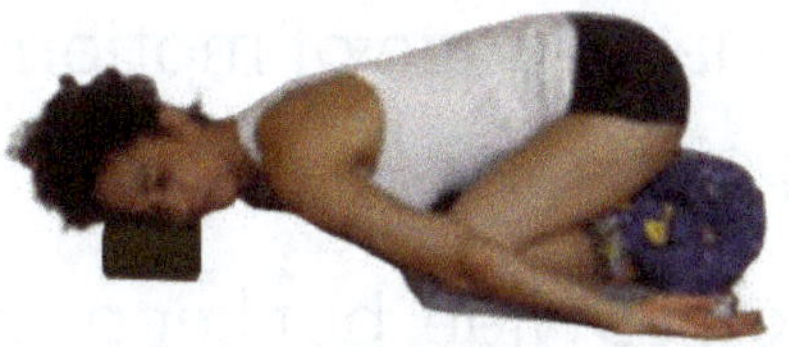

Variation C: Child Pose with Block and Arms Bent

This variation is easier on the shoulders.

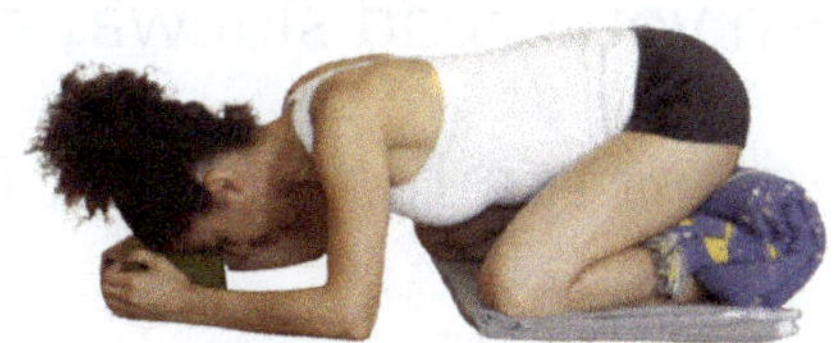

BENEFITS

The child's pose calms the mind, relieves stress, opens up the hips, and stretches the inner thighs, lower back, and ankles. This specific variation opens and stretches the shoulders. If this is uncomfortable or you have tight shoulders, try variation B.

SET UP

- Fold a blanket under your knees for comfort
- Get on all fours with your lower legs on a folded blanket
- Fold or roll another blanket and place it behind your knees. If you lack range of motion at this joint, this will relieve the pain.
- Open your knees wide, but keep your big toes together
- Rest your forehead on a block or extra firm pillow.
- Extend your arms forward (Extended Child Pose with Block) or toward your feet (Extend Child Pose with block facing sideways). If your arms extend toward your feet, turn your head sideways.
- Slow down your breath and relax for five minutes or longer.

BASIC CHILD POSE VARIATIONS

Variation A: Extended Child Pose with arms extended.

This variation opens and stretches the shoulders. If this is uncomfortable or you have tight shoulders, try variation B.

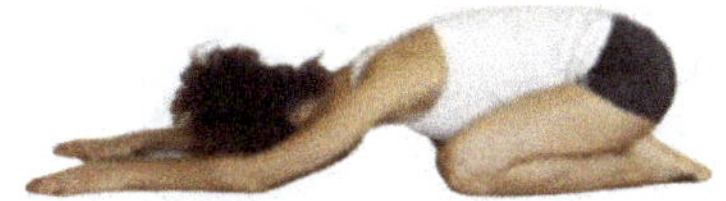

Variation B: Child Pose with Arms Extended Toward The Feet.

This variation is easier on the shoulders.

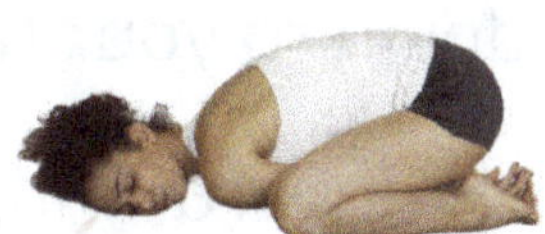

Variation C: Child Pose with Arms Between The Knees.

This variation provides a deeper stretch in the hips, spine, and shoulders and can feel more intense.

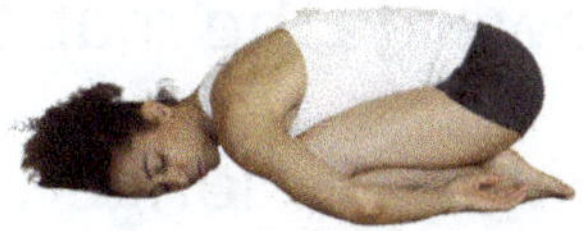

BENEFITS

These Child's Pose variations require the most mobility in the hips and shoulders because there are no props involved; Child's Pose variations calm the mind, relieve stress, open up the hips, stretch the inner thighs, lengthen the back muscles and ankles. It promotes digestion and increases blood flow to the head.

INSTRUCTIONS

- Start on all fours on your yoga mat
- Open your knees wide and keep your big toes together
- Bring your hips down to your heels
- Walk your hands forward until your elbows are fully extended. Alternatively, experiment with reaching your arms toward your feet or even between your knees. Notice how each variation feels different.
- Bring your chest close to the floor.
- Place your forehead on your yoga mat or towel. Your face can face towards the mat or sideways.
- Rest for five minutes or longer.

CHAPTER 8

SEATED FORWARD FOLD VARIATIONS

LOTUS POSE

⚠ **WARNING**

This is an advanced pose that requires some degree of hip flexibility. If you experience discomfort in your knees while settling into this pose, your hips are not ready for this pose yet. Gently ease out and select another pose.

This pose requires deep hip and spine flexibility. Only attempt it once the previous childpose variations feel comfortable for you.

LOTUS POSE

Option A: Supported Lotus Pose with bolster and blocks.

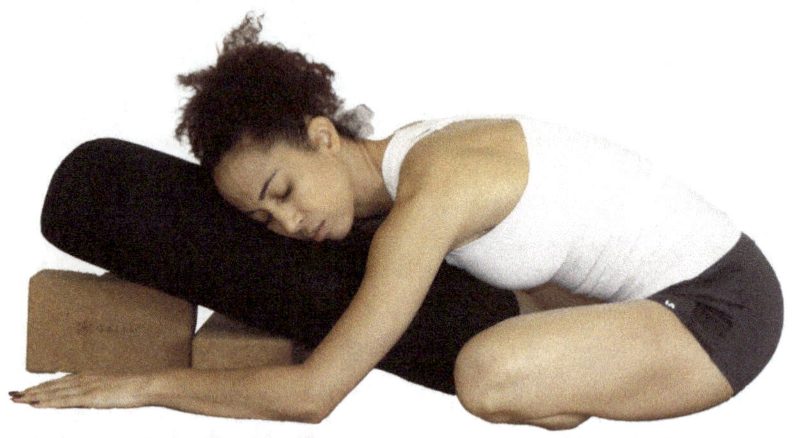

Option B: Supported Lotus Pose with pillows and towels.

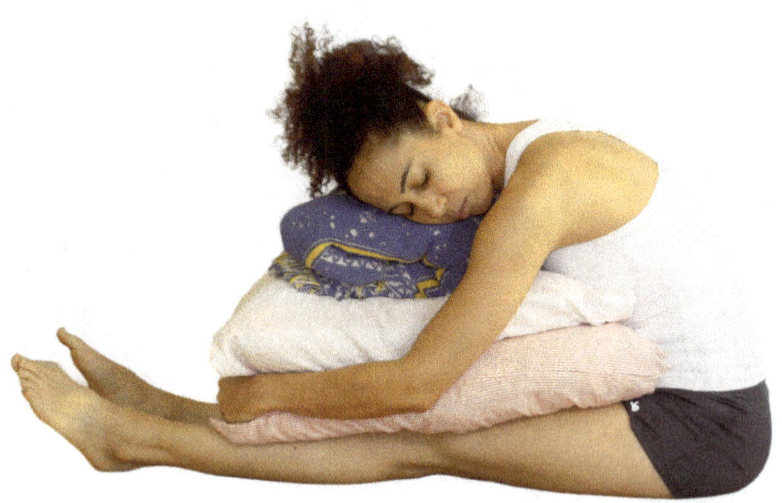

BENEFITS

Lotus Pose opens up the hips, stretches the inner things, lengthens the back muscles, and helps develop good posture. Additionally, this pose promotes mental awareness and calms the nervous system.

SET UP

- Start by setting up your blocks. First, place the block furthest away on one of its small surfaces to create the incline.
- Place the block closer to you on its wider surface.
- Place your bolster over the blocks to create the incline.
- Sit with your legs crossed in a lotus position.
- Bend at the crease of your hips to fold forward. Aim at maintaining a smooth curve in the spine.
- Lay your abdomen on the bolster and relax for five minutes or longer.

TIPS

1) Add a large pillow at the base of the bolster for extra support. This can be useful if your hips and lower back are tight.

2) If you do not have a bolster, use large firm pillows and blankets. Fold them so they are snug under your abdomen when you lean forward (option B).

SUPPORTED SEATED FORWARD FOLD

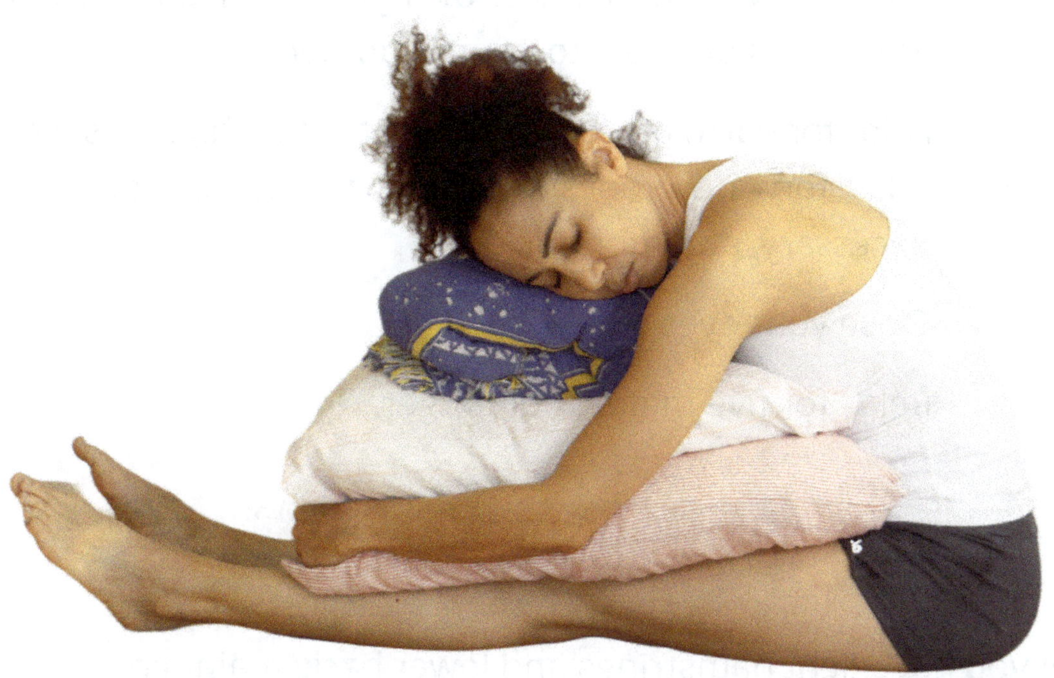

BENEFITS

Seated forward folds calm the mind, soothe the nervous system, alleviate anxiety, and reduce fatigue and insomnia. This pose also stretches the hamstrings, calves, and lower back muscles. It can also help improve symptoms of menopause and menstrual discomfort.

SET UP

- Sit up on your mat and extend your legs. Fold large, firm pillows and blankets over your thighs. Pull them as close as possible to your abdomen.
- Fold forward at the crease of your hips. As you relax forward, you should feel totally supported. If necessary, add more pillows.
- Close your eyes
- Relax for five minutes or longer.

TIPS

If you have tight hamstrings and lower back, maintain a slight knee bent. You can roll a large towel underneath your knees to provide support. Additionally, you can fold a large towel and place it under your hips. This will make it easier to bend forward.

SEATED STRADDLE

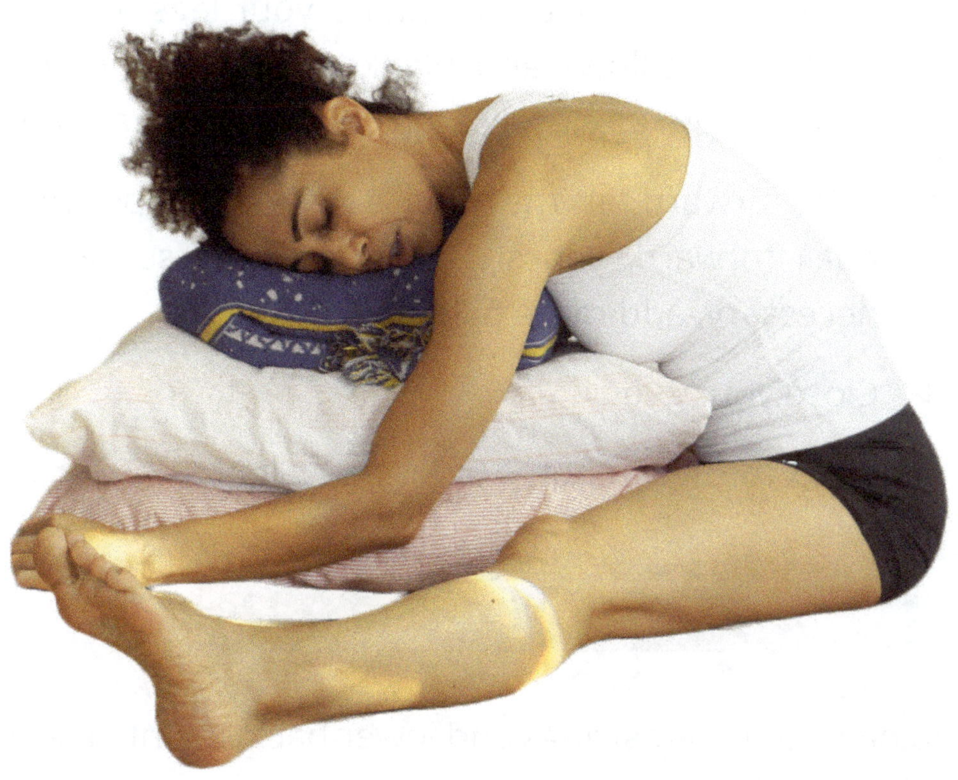

BENEFITS

The straddle pose calms the mind, soothes the nervous system, alleviates anxiety, and reduces fatigue and insomnia. This pose also stretches the hamstrings, inner thigh muscles, and lower back muscles and opens the hips. It can also improve symptoms of menopause and menstrual discomfort.

SET UP

- Sit up on your mat and extend your legs wide open. Fold large pillows and blankets between your legs, and ull them as closely as possible to your abdomen.
- Fold forward at the crease of your hips. As you relax forward, you should feel totally supported. If necessary, add more pillows.
- Close your eyes
- Relax for five minutes or longer.

TIP

If you have tight hamstrings and lower back, maintain a slight knee bend. Additionally, you can fold a large towel and place it under your hips, making it easier to bend forward.

CHAPTER 9

UPPER BACK AND SHOULDER RELIEF

SAVASANA VARIATIONS

In this chapter, you will receive several variations of the same pose. They each offer a different feel, comfort, and intensity. Try them all to figure out which one suits you the most.

Savasana poses calm the nervous system, relax the mind, and ease stress, fatigue, and anxiety. Savasana also helps lower blood pressure. They have a meditative effect and promote spiritual awakening.

SAVASANA WITH BOLSTER

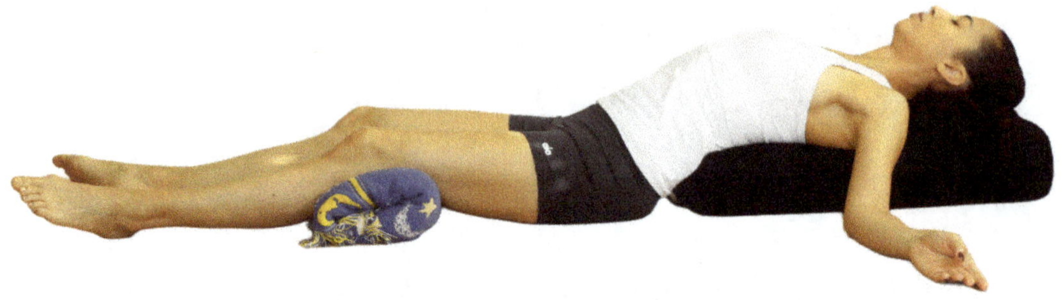

BENEFITS

These heart openers stretch the chest muscles and shoulder joint, open up the upper back, and facilitate deep breathing. They relieve tired, achy lower and upper backs and help improve posture.

SET UP

- Sit up with your hips close to your bolster
- Roll a blanket and place it under your knees. This takes the pressure off your lower back.
- Sit in front of your bolster
- Lay back on your bolster, keeping the hips on your mat. The end of the bolster should snug the arch of your lower back to provide support.
- Open your arms sideways. You may feel a deep stretch in your chest and shoulders.
- Close your eyes
- Relax for five minutes or longer

SAVASANA WITH BLOCKS

Variation A: Savasana with blocks horizontal.

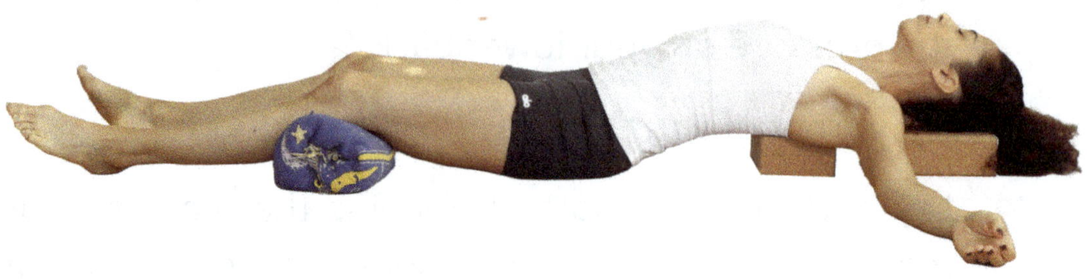

Variation B: Savasana with blocks vertical.

Choose this option if you want to deepen the sensation in the back.

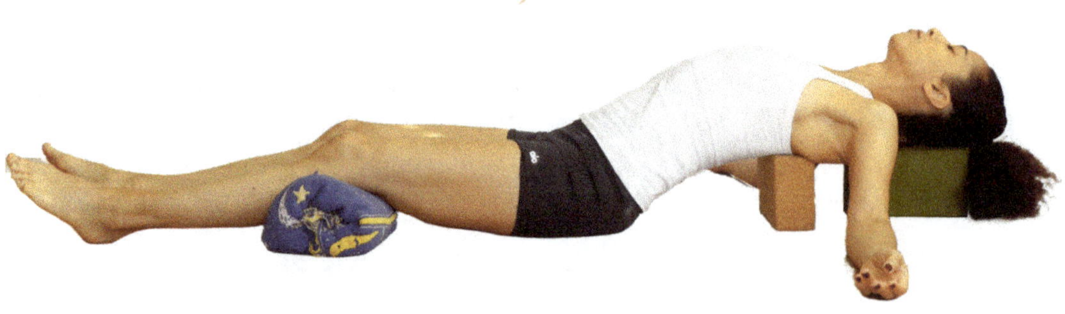

BENEFITS

These variations of Savasana stretch the chest muscles and shoulder joint, open up the upper back, and facilitate deep breathing. It provides relief for tired, achy upper backs.

SET UP

- Start by setting up your blocks in a T-shape.
- Sit up on your yoga mat
- Roll a blanket and place it under your knees. This will take the pressure off your lower back.
- Lay back so that the bottom block supports your shoulder blades and the upper block supports your head
- Open your arms sideways
- Close your eyes
- Relax for five minutes or longer.

SAVASANA WITH BOLSTER AND BLOCK

Variations A: Bending the knees or placing a pillow underneath the knees relieves lower back tension.

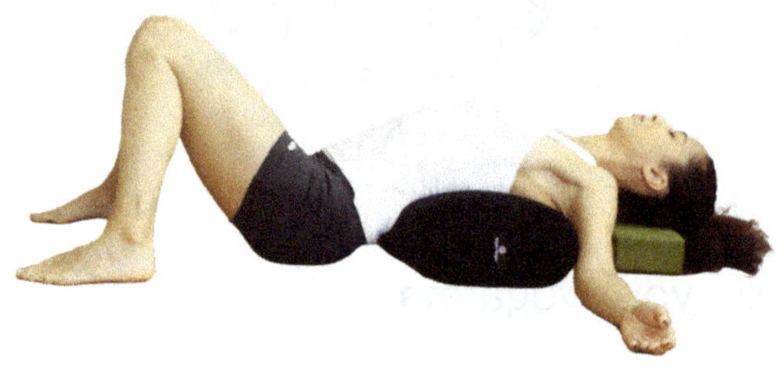

Variation B: Savasana with bolster and block with legs supported. The pillow underneath the knees relieves the pressure in the lower back.

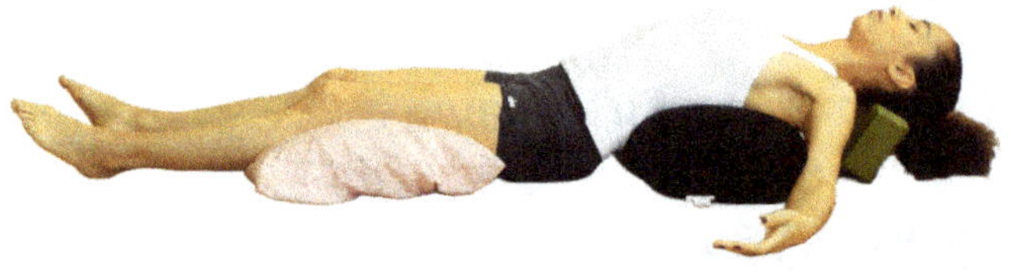

Variation C: Savasana with knees extended.

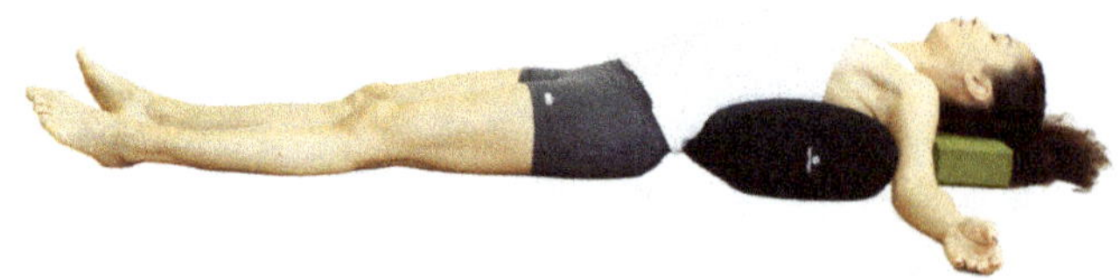

BENEFITS

Savasana stretches the chest muscles and shoulder joint, open up the upper back, and facilitates deep breathing. They provide relief for tired, achy upper backs. These variations offer a deep stretch in the chest and shoulders, promoting improved posture and upper back and neck relief.

SET UP

- Start by setting up your bolster perpendicular to the direction of your yoga mat
- Place your block a few inches away from your bolster
- Sit up on your yoga mat
- Optional: Bend your knees or roll a blanket and place it under your knees
- Lay back so that your bolster supports your shoulder blades and the block supports your head
- Open your arms sideways and notice the release in your chest and shoulders
- Close your eyes
- Relax for five minutes or longer

SUPINE BUTTERFLY

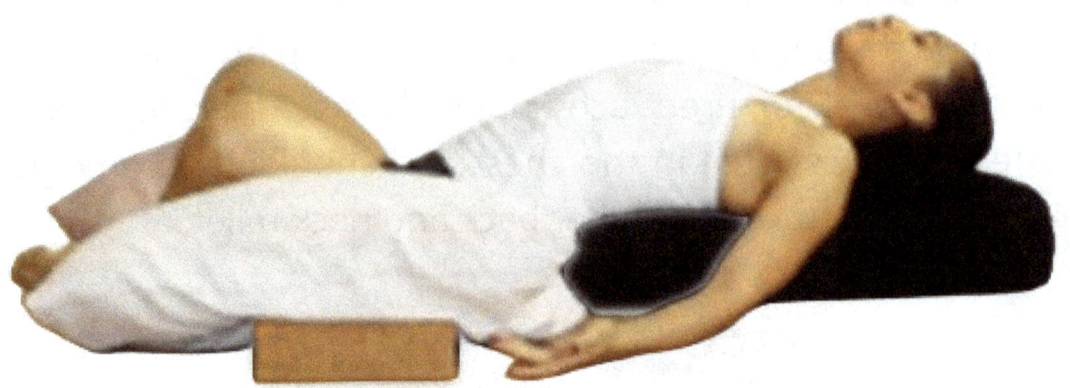

BENEFITS

Butterfly Pose loosens your lower back and hips and stretches your inner thighs. The bolster provides relief for the chest and shoulders. This pose has a calming and meditative effect on the nervous system. This restorative pose helps ease joint discomfort.

SET UP

- Sit on the floor
- Place your bolster lengthwise behind your tailbone
- Place your legs in butterfly with your knees bent and the soles of your feet against one another
- Place the blocks under your thighs
- Optional: Place one pillow on each block for more comfort.
- Rest and relax for five minutes or longer.

CHAPTER 10

EXPLORING ADDITIONAL PATHS OF RELIEF

WALL STRADDLE

This advanced stretch requires hip and shoulder range of motion and flexibility in the inner thighs. It may not be suitable at the beginner's stage. However, the blocks help make the pose more accessible for individuals with limited inner thigh flexibility.

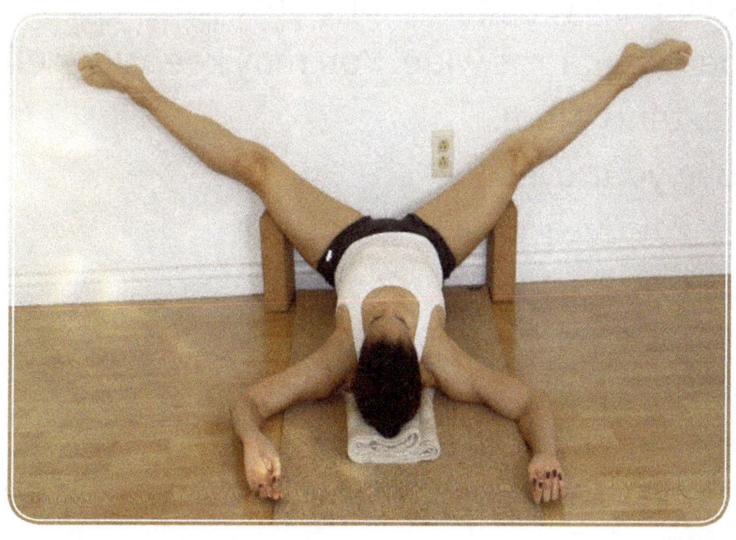

BENEFITS

The wall straddle opens the hips, stretches the inner thighs, and releases lower back tension. The arms above the head help open the chest, upper back, and shoulder joints. This restorative pose reduces anxiety and stress. It is also known to ease symptoms of menopause and PMS.

SET UP

- Fold a blanket perpendicular to the wall
- Sit sideways with your right hip close to the wall
- Swing your legs up against the wall as you lay on your blanket
- Scoop your hips as close to the wall as possible
- Spread your legs wide open
- Use blocks to support and rest your legs
- Open your arms wide. You may keep your elbows bent or extend them.
- Close your eyes
- Rest for five minutes or longer.

TIPS

Scoop your hips away from the wall if this pose is challenging.

SUPINE TWIST

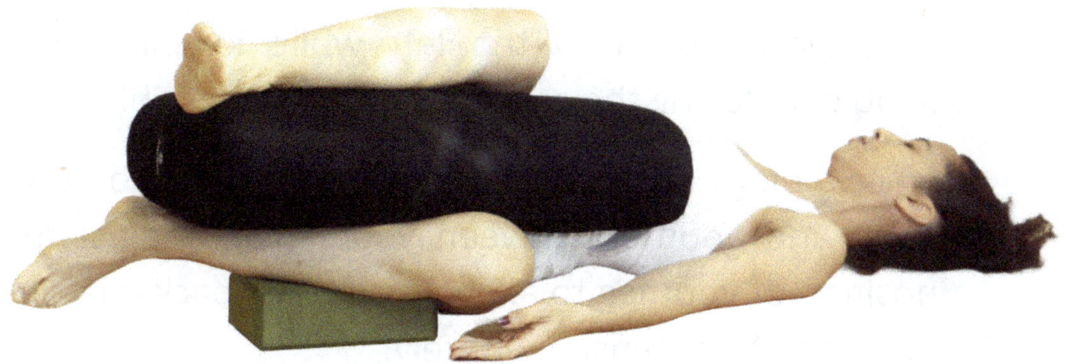

BENEFITS

Supine twists help reduce bloating, improve digestion, and relieve tight lower back and shoulder muscles. It also helps relieve lower back and hip pain and improve spine mobility.

SET UP

- Lay on your back with your knees bent
- Drop your knees to the left while keeping your shoulders facing the ceiling as much as possible.
- Place a block, bolster, or pillow(s) under your bottom thigh and another between your knees. Adjust the position of your leg to allow your lower back muscles to let go of any tension entirely.
- Press your right shoulder against the floor.
- Tilt your chin to the right or keep it facing straight up.
- Close your eyes and relax for five minutes or more.

SIDE SNUGGLE

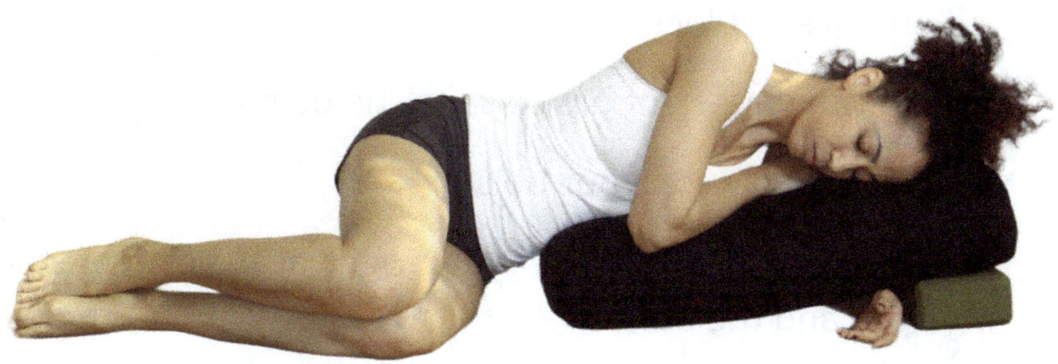

BENEFITS

Side Snuggle relieves lower back pressure, reduces mental tension, and promotes a sense of calm.

SET UP

- Place your bolster lengthwise on your mat with one end over a block
- Sit with your right hip close to the bolster
- Lay sideways on your bolster
- Snug your bolster with your right arm between the floor and the bolster
- Close your eyes
- Relax for five minutes or longer

CHAPTER 11

CONCLUSION

In "5-Minute Restorative Yoga Stretches for Seniors over 60," you have discovered an invaluable resource for revitalizing your mind, body, and spirit. The book offers a comprehensive collection of gentle exercises you can return to anytime to ease stress and anxiety and promote pain-free joints. As you embark on this journey, it is essential to recognize that the benefits of these exercises take time to manifest and deepen. Regular, consistent practice is critical to unlocking their full potential.

Consider this book not the end of an accomplishment but rather a starting point, a gateway to a healthier and more balanced lifestyle. As you continue to immerse yourself in the 15-minute restorative yoga stretches, you will gradually experience their transformative power. With each session, you will notice an improvement in your range of motion, with less strain on your muscles. It is through dedication and perseverance that the true benefits unfold. Embrace this book as a stepping stone, and let it empower you to take charge of your health.

Personalized training can additionally be immensely beneficial for a more tailored approach and accelerated results. By seeking personalized guidance, you can receive individualized instructions, exercises, and programs that cater to your unique needs and goals. To explore this option further, schedule a 15-Minute FREE Discovery Session with me by typing the URL in your web browser.

Schedule a 15-Minute Free Discovery Session: https://qr1.be/C6CP

Alternatively, you can point your phone camera to the QR code below and tap the screen to be directed to the scheduling page. This will redirect you to a page to **schedule a 15-Minute FREE discovery session** with me. During this session, we will explore your struggles, past experiences, goals, and options.

15-Minute Free Discovery Session QR CODE

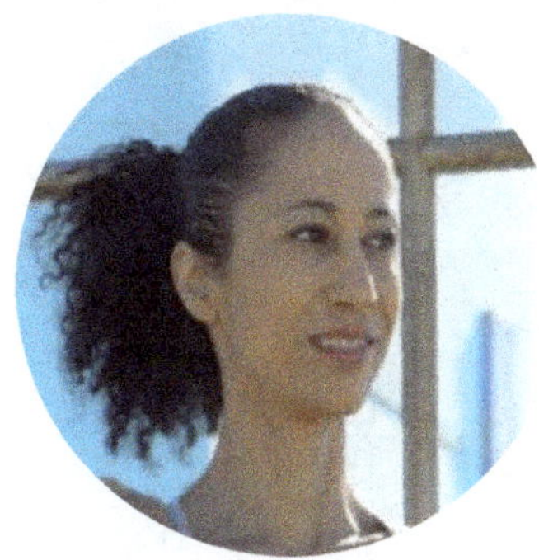

If you enjoyed this book, please support me by leaving a review, suggesting it to your friends and family, or offering it as a gift; it only takes minutes.

To share a review, point your phone's camera at the QR code below and tap the camera on the screen.

QR CODE FOR REVIEW

www.ingramcontent.com/pod-product-compliance
Lightning Source LLC
LaVergne TN
LVHW081320110826
845149LV00006B/1554

9798988544005